THE THERAPY JOURNAL
A Guided Reflection Space for Therapy Sessions

Designed by therapists to help you
get the most out of therapy.

. . . .

(THIS BOOK BELONGS TO)

. . . .

(IF FOUND, PLEASE RETURN TO)

LEARN MORE
www.therapynotebooks.com

THERAPY NOTEBOOKS
Published by Subject Matters

ISBN: 9781958963975
Printed in the United States of America

LEAD THERAPISTS
Diana Hu, PsyD
Kathleen Maher, LCSW

EDITED BY
Alexandra Ossola
Hod Tamir, PhD

DESIGNED BY
Monumento.Co

BRANDING BY
High Tide

IF YOU ARE IN URGENT
NEED OF ASSISTANCE:
Dial 9-1-1

FOR MENTAL HEALTH
CRISIS SUPPORT:
Dial 9-8-8

SAMHSA National Helpline
1-800-622-HELP (4357)

Crisis Text Line
Text HOME to 741741

Letter From a Therapist

As a clinician, I know that being here means you've already taken an important step on your mental health journey. Seeking therapy means that you want to make a change—maybe you want more insight into your behavior, to forge better connections with others, or just a time outside your normal day-to-day to process your emotions. You've navigated the logistical hurdles to finding a therapist and showed up with the optimism that a clinician will be able to help you. That takes courage, vulnerability, and more than a little hope.

But even so, questions may come up for you. "Does my therapist understand me?" "Are they the right fit?" "Do they have an approach that will work for me?" And, perhaps most importantly, "Will I make progress?"

These are understandable worries, ones that I often hear from the clients who come through my door. These concerns can show up as clients' reluctance to share openly about their lives. It can take time to get to know each other, and the fear of being misunderstood or misrepresented is palpable. Other times, they may feel sensitive as we dig into the root cause of what brought them into therapy. I recognize and appreciate these reactions— trust comes with the push and pull of getting to know each other. Often, clients have lived with a problem for a long time, and it can be stressful, or even threatening, to try to resolve it.

Unlike other forms of care, therapy is rooted in lived, human experience—it's nuanced, complex, and emotional. There is no one-size-fits-all treatment that works for everyone and, even more frustratingly, there is no guarantee for success at the outset. This can feel daunting. Therapy is also unique in what it asks of you. Not only is the work emotionally impactful—you may be identifying sensitive or painful areas of your life—but it also requires you to be highly engaged. Your therapist may assign you homework, ask you to reflect on important questions, and actively make changes in your life to see progress. Finding time and mental space for that work can be a challenge in and of itself.

We created this journal to be a helpful tool as you navigate the intricacies, challenges, and successes of therapy. It will give you the structure and space to figure out what you'd like to change, to emotionally prepare to share openly with your therapist, and to incorporate learnings from sessions into your life as you assess how they're working for you. We hope this companion makes your courageous next step a little easier.

Sincerely,

Diana Hu, PsyD, with support from
Kathleen Maher, LCSW
Lead Clinicians

Scan the QR code to
meet our clinicians

How This Book Helps You

1 Get the most out of your therapy sessions.

Instead of wondering whether or not therapy "works" for you, enjoy the feeling of tangible progress. This notebook is designed to help you get clear about what you want out of therapy, and how to focus your sessions so you're making the most of them.

2 Explore the therapist-approved system designed for before, during, and after your sessions.

This journal offers a unique blend of structure and flexibility to help you capture and explore 20 complete sessions of therapy—whether you're just starting out, resuming after a while, or are well on the way to transformation.

3 Never draw a blank in session again.

We'll help you prioritize topics and highlight discoveries between sessions so that you're prepared to talk about what matters most to you.

4 Bring your therapy insights to life.

So much of our healing takes place outside of therapy. Whether it's completing homework, cataloging observations, or making time to reflect, your notebook will help you take your work off the couch and into the world.

5 Made by therapists who understand how challenging therapy can be.

The therapists behind this journal have extensive experience supporting their clients in challenging emotional work. They've designed this notebook to give you the framework you need to chart a clear path forward.

Contents

INTRODUCTION:
Collaboration at the Heart of Therapy

You've started therapy because you want to make a change. That's within reach—decades of research have identified the factors that contribute to successful therapy and, in turn, improved outcomes for clients.[1] These include differences in treatment decisions, the therapist's ability to empathize with the client, their sensitivity to the client's cultural background, how the therapist shares about themselves, and the client's expectations and attitudes toward therapy.[2]

But the most important factor, studies have found, hinges on the therapist-client relationship. In a strong therapist-client relationship, the client trusts the therapist enough to speak openly and vulnerably, and to share their inner thoughts, even if it is not easy.[3] Neither the therapist nor the client dominates this relationship, but each takes turns leading and following.[4] Both respect one another, are empathetic, and assume the other's best intentions.

Experts often call this working relationship the "therapeutic alliance."[5] In a 2006 study, researchers Robert Hatcher and Alex Barends describe the therapeutic alliance as "the degree to which the therapy [pair] is engaged in collaborative, purposive work."[6] In a strong alliance, the client and therapist have a positive relationship, they agree on the goals of their work together, and are aligned on what tasks or methods the therapy will entail.

Working together on goals and approach to care creates rapport between client and therapist so that the client feels comfortable sharing details with the therapist that might be helpful in treatment. The therapist, in the meantime, supports and validates the client, giving them space to address more immediate issues as they come up while also keeping their goals in mind. Even imperfect moments—for example, when the therapist didn't react with total support, or the client didn't take feedback well—can be opportunities to strengthen the relationship.[7]

Put another way, as a client, you can influence the outcomes of therapy through collaboration and intentional engagement with your therapist. Your active participation can help build a strong therapeutic alliance.

This journal is set up to help foster that critical collaboration between you and your therapist. It's designed to help you use your time outside your sessions so that the sessions themselves are even more impactful.

Here are some of the ways this journal can support, and, hopefully, improve your therapy experience:

SET YOUR GOAL FOR THERAPY

Identify what progress will look like for you by setting a "north star" for therapy. This is typically something you would set with your therapist and refine over time as you test and learn. You'll periodically check in on your goals and your therapist relationship to make sure they're still working for you.

REFLECT ON YOUR WEEK WITH GUIDED PROMPTS

Before your session, capture the key moments and thought patterns that you'd like to unpack with your therapist. Organize your thoughts so you can share whatever is most pressing to you. The prompts change every week so you can choose what kind of reflection resonates most.

PREPARE INTENTIONALLY TO BE FULLY PRESENT FOR YOUR SESSION

You might be going to therapy after a tough day of work or after a stressful conversation with your partner. Life happens, and it can be hard to engage in something as participatory as therapy when you're still preoccupied by something that just happened. You might also need to mindfully pause before transitioning into "therapy mode." We created a pre-session check-in for you to understand how you're feeling and whether you'd like to discuss it with your therapist during the session.

CAPTURE YOUR THERAPY INSIGHTS IN
REAL-TIME WITH NOTES AND TAKEAWAYS

You or your therapist might have said something—a phrase, a term, an observation—that really resonated with you. We've provided dedicated space for you to process your session as it's happening, and capture the key insights that you'd like to reflect on after the session's end.

PROCESS YOUR SESSION AND PUT IT INTO ACTION

A therapy session can feel short, yet incredibly emotionally impactful. Immediately after the session, get started on your post-session work by continuing the reflection with guided prompts. Jot down anything you've missed or anything you'd like to translate into action for your upcoming week.

A strong therapeutic relationship can help you see the change you've been hoping for. That said, it's important to recognize if you and your therapist don't seem to be working well together. Find tips for adjusting your therapy or finding a therapist who's a better fit in Appendix D.

Good luck, and happy collaborating.

How This Journal Works

This journal is designed to fit seamlessly into your therapy journey. Each session entry will empower you to reflect and integrate the insights you've gained from your sessions. While we created this journal with weekly sessions in mind, you can easily adjust your use based on your therapy schedule. As always, use this journal in a way that best suits you.

WHAT IT HELPS YOU DO	HOW IT HELPS	SUGGESTED USE*
Set your goals for therapy.	Set your goals at the start of journal, and check in at the middle and end to help you establish and clarify your goals.	Every 2-3 months.
Reflect on your week.	Journaling space with guided prompts to encourage you to reflect on key events, thoughts, and feelings.	Daily, leading up to the session.
Prepare intentionally for session.	Pre-session check-in to mindfully transition from busyness to session readiness.	Shortly before the session.
Capture your therapy insights in real time.	Dedicated space to take notes from your session.	During the session.
Process your session and put it into action.	Guided reflection space to continue integrating what you've learned.	Shortly after the session.

* "Suggested use" is our recommendation for when each feature would best be used, but you should ultimately do what works best for you.

Setting Your Goal

Note From
a Therapist

Establishing a therapy goal ensures that you and your therapist
are on the same page about the focus of the work and what
progress looks like. Once you've figured out a goal, your therapist
will suggest a plan intended to help you move towards it.

Because goal-setting is so central to therapy, and because
it can be hard to pinpoint that goal on your own, we've created
a guided exercise to help you do that. You'll check in every few
months to refine your goal as you progress through therapy.

Here are *key questions* that will help you set a therapy goal:

1   What is the broad issue that brings you to therapy?

This is often a change you would like to make in your life, such
as, *"I want to feel less depressed."* Do your best to name that issue
and what you'd like to change.

2   How is it affecting you?

This is the reason for wanting to change. *For example*, if you were
less depressed, what would you be able to do?

3   What are the barriers to change?

Change can be hard, even if it's for the better. We may know that
something isn't working, but can still feel reluctant to change

because of mental, emotional, or logistical barriers. Understanding yours can help you overcome them. Continuing with our example, perhaps you feel a sense of hopelessness that makes you believe that if you try anything new, you'll only fail.

All together, your therapy goal should address the barriers that keep you from making the changes you want. Your goal could be something like, *"I want to address my sense of hopelessness so that I can feel connected with my hobbies and friends again."*

Reflect

1   What is the broad issue that brings you to therapy?

Example: i feel really anxious and have panic attacks.

2   How is it affecting you? What would you be able to do if it were resolved?

Example: I wish I could go out and feel more comfortable just being out, and not waiting to see if

I'll get anxious and break down in panic. I'd like to actually be able to enjoy myself!

3   What are the barriers to change?

Example: I don't know how to get my thoughts to slow down, or if my fears are justified. I'm also

worried that I won't be able to make it better even if I try.

Set Your Goal

Example: My goal is to be less anxious and have fewer panic attacks by learning how

to slow down my thoughts, check my fears against reality, and manage my worries.

Then, I can feel more comfortable in public without being hyper-alert to anxiety or panic.

Reflect

1   What is the broad issue that brings you to therapy?

2   How is it affecting you? What would you be able to do if it were resolved?

3   What are the barriers to change?

         Set Your Goal

Session 01

Use the next two pages to free write, or choose any of the prompts below to help you get started—whatever is most helpful for you to process and reflect in preparation for your session.

WRITING PROMPTS

- What is something you noticed recently that you haven't noticed before?

- What is a "win" that you'd like to share with your therapist?

- What was the most pervasive or "sticky" thought that you've had?

M | D | Y |

M | D | Y |

M | D | Y |

M | D | Y |

M | D | Y |

M | D | Y |

Session Preparation

Take a few deep breaths. Imagine turning down the volume on all the "noise" of your day. Try to actively disconnect from any distractions, including devices, emails, or to-do lists (refer to Appendix A for Mindfulness Techniques).

When you feel ready, let's check in before your therapy session.

Pre-Session Check-In

How are you feeling right now?

(0)—(1)—(2)—(3)—(4)—(5)—(6)—(7)—(8)—(9)—(10)

TERRIBLE   AMAZING

1   What thoughts, emotions, or physical sensations do you notice right now?
       You can refer to The Feelings Wheel in Appendix B for help naming the emotions.

2   What is contributing to how you're feeling?

Topics for This Session

What are your priorities for this session? This may include what you're currently feeling, topics from your Notes From the Week, and/or the goals you set for therapy.

1

2

3

Session Notes

Jot down helpful notes and highlights from your therapy session.

Key Takeaways

Capture the learnings, insights, and/or action items from the therapy session.

1

2

3

Session Reflection

Continue to reflect on your session, what you've learned, and how you want to incorporate these insights into your day-to-day life.

1   How are you feeling? Were there any thoughts or ideas that stood out to you?

2   Were there topics that you didn't get to in this session or wish you could have kept talking about?

3   How would you like to incorporate the takeaways you noted during the session into your week?

Session 02

Use the next two pages to free write, or choose any of the
prompts below to help you get started—whatever is most helpful
for you to process and reflect in preparation for your session.

WRITING PROMPTS

- What thoughts or feelings did you notice having today?

- How do you know when you're feeling vulnerable?

- What was your favorite moment today?

M | D | Y |

M | D | Y |

M | D | Y |

M | D | Y |

M | D | Y |

M | D | Y |

Session Preparation

Take a few deep breaths. Imagine turning down the volume on all the "noise" of your day. Try to actively disconnect from any distractions, including devices, emails, or to-do lists (refer to Appendix A for Mindfulness Techniques).

When you feel ready, let's check in before your therapy session.

Pre-Session Check-In

How are you feeling right now?

(0)—(1)—(2)—(3)—(4)—(5)—(6)—(7)—(8)—(9)—(10)

TERRIBLE   AMAZING

1   What thoughts, emotions, or physical sensations do you notice right now?
    You can refer to The Feelings Wheel in Appendix B for help naming the emotions.

2   What is contributing to how you're feeling?

Topics for This Session

What are your priorities for this session? This may include what you're currently feeling, topics from your Notes From the Week, and/or the goals you set for therapy.

1

2

3

Session Notes

Jot down helpful notes and highlights from your therapy session.

Key Takeaways

Capture the learnings, insights, and/or action items from the therapy session.

1

2

3

Session Reflection

Continue to reflect on your session, what you've learned, and how you want to incorporate these insights into your day-to-day life.

1   How are you feeling? Were there any thoughts or ideas that stood out to you?

2   Were there topics that you didn't get to in this session or wish you could have kept talking about?

3   How would you like to incorporate the takeaways you noted during the session into your week?

Session 03

Use the next two pages to free write, or choose any of the prompts below to help you get started—whatever is most helpful for you to process and reflect in preparation for your session.

WRITING PROMPTS

- If you were to make a pie chart of the feelings you've experienced so far this week, what would it look like?

- What is a relationship that you would like to foster?

- How do you think you've been doing in dealing with life stressors recently?

M | D | Y |

M | D | Y |

M | D | Y |

M | D | Y |

M | D | Y |

M | D | Y |

Session Preparation

Take a few deep breaths. Imagine turning down the volume on all the "noise" of your day. Try to actively disconnect from any distractions, including devices, emails, or to-do lists (refer to Appendix A for Mindfulness Techniques).

When you feel ready, let's check in before your therapy session.

Pre-Session Check-In

How are you feeling right now?

(0)—(1)—(2)—(3)—(4)—(5)—(6)—(7)—(8)—(9)—(10)

TERRIBLE   AMAZING

What thoughts, emotions, or physical sensations do you notice right now?
You can refer to The Feelings Wheel in Appendix B for help naming the emotions.

What is contributing to how you're feeling?

Topics for This Session

What are your priorities for this session? This may include what you're currently feeling, topics from your Notes From the Week, and/or the goals you set for therapy.

1

2

3

Session Notes

Jot down helpful notes and highlights from your therapy session.

Key Takeaways

Capture the learnings, insights, and/or action items from the therapy session.

Session Reflection

Continue to reflect on your session, what you've learned, and how you want to incorporate these insights into your day-to-day life.

1   How are you feeling? Were there any thoughts or ideas that stood out to you?

2   Were there topics that you didn't get to in this session or wish you could have kept
         talking about?

3   How would you like to incorporate the takeaways you noted during the session
         into your week?

Session 04

Use the next two pages to free write, or choose any of the prompts below to help you get started—whatever is most helpful for you to process and reflect in preparation for your session.

WRITING PROMPTS

- What boundaries did you notice being set today, by yourself or others?

- What is something you've done to get out of your comfort zone?

- What is something you noticed today that you feel grateful for?

M | D | Y |

M | D | Y |

M | D | Y |

M | D | Y

M | D | Y

M | D | Y

Session Preparation

Take a few deep breaths. Imagine turning down the volume on all the "noise" of your day. Try to actively disconnect from any distractions, including devices, emails, or to-do lists (refer to Appendix A for Mindfulness Techniques).

When you feel ready, let's check in before your therapy session.

Pre-Session Check-In

How are you feeling right now?

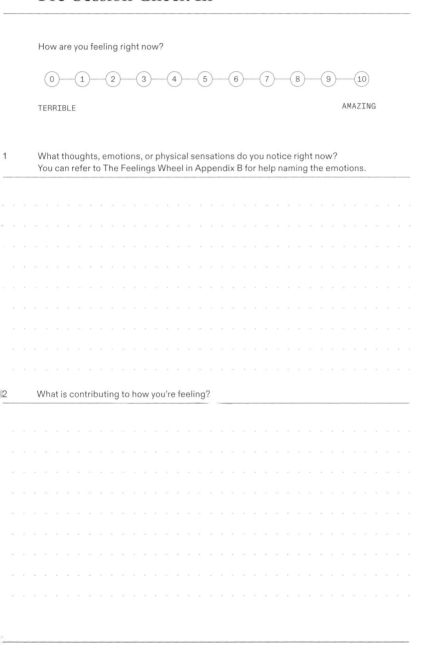

TERRIBLE   AMAZING

---

1   What thoughts, emotions, or physical sensations do you notice right now?
     You can refer to The Feelings Wheel in Appendix B for help naming the emotions.

2   What is contributing to how you're feeling?

Topics for This Session

What are your priorities for this session? This may include what you're currently feeling, topics from your Notes From the Week, and/or the goals you set for therapy.

1

2

3

Session Notes

Jot down helpful notes and highlights from your therapy session.

Key Takeaways

Capture the learnings, insights, and/or action items from the therapy session.

1

2

3

Session Reflection

Continue to reflect on your session, what you've learned, and how you want to incorporate these insights into your day-to-day life.

1   How are you feeling? Were there any thoughts or ideas that stood out to you?

2   Were there topics that you didn't get to in this session or wish you could have kept talking about?

3   How would you like to incorporate the takeaways you noted during the session into your week?

Session 05

Use the next two pages to free write, or choose any of the
prompts below to help you get started—whatever is most helpful
for you to process and reflect in preparation for your session.

WRITING PROMPTS

- What is something you did differently recently than you
  have in the past?

- Is there a thought about a feeling or event that keeps
  coming back to you? What is that thought?

- When did you recently feel really connected to and in-tune
  with your body?

M | D | Y |

M | D | Y |

M | D | Y |

| D | Y | |

| D | Y | |

| D | Y | |

Session Preparation

Take a few deep breaths. Imagine turning down the volume on all the "noise" of your day. Try to actively disconnect from any distractions, including devices, emails, or to-do lists (refer to Appendix A for Mindfulness Techniques).

When you feel ready, let's check in before your therapy session.

Pre-Session Check-In

How are you feeling right now?

(0)—(1)—(2)—(3)—(4)—(5)—(6)—(7)—(8)—(9)—(10)

TERRIBLE   AMAZING

1   What thoughts, emotions, or physical sensations do you notice right now?
     You can refer to The Feelings Wheel in Appendix B for help naming the emotions.

2   What is contributing to how you're feeling?

Topics for This Session

What are your priorities for this session? This may include what you're currently feeling, topics from your Notes From the Week, and/or the goals you set for therapy.

1

2

3

Session Notes

Jot down helpful notes and highlights from your therapy session.

Key Takeaways

Capture the learnings, insights, and/or action items from the therapy session.

Session Reflection

Continue to reflect on your session, what you've learned, and how you want to incorporate these insights into your day-to-day life.

1   How are you feeling? Were there any thoughts or ideas that stood out to you?

2   Were there topics that you didn't get to in this session or wish you could have kept talking about?

3   How would you like to incorporate the takeaways you noted during the session into your week?

Session 06

Use the next two pages to free write, or choose any of the prompts below to help you get started—whatever is most helpful for you to process and reflect in preparation for your session.

WRITING PROMPTS

- What do you feel most worried or anxious about?

- How did you see one of your strengths playing out today?

- What was the strongest feeling you had today?

M | D | Y |

M | D | Y |

M | D | Y |

M | D | Y |

M | D | Y |

M | D | Y |

Session Preparation

Take a few deep breaths. Imagine turning down the volume on all the "noise" of your day. Try to actively disconnect from any distractions, including devices, emails, or to-do lists (refer to Appendix A for Mindfulness Techniques).

When you feel ready, let's check in before your therapy session.

Pre-Session Check-In

How are you feeling right now?

(0)—(1)—(2)—(3)—(4)—(5)—(6)—(7)—(8)—(9)—(10)

TERRIBLE   AMAZING

1   What thoughts, emotions, or physical sensations do you notice right now?
    You can refer to The Feelings Wheel in Appendix B for help naming the emotions.

2   What is contributing to how you're feeling?

Topics for This Session

What are your priorities for this session? This may include what you're currently feeling, topics from your Notes From the Week, and/or the goals you set for therapy.

1

2

3

Session Notes

Jot down helpful notes and highlights from your therapy session.

Key Takeaways

Capture the learnings, insights, and/or action items from the therapy session.

Session Reflection

Continue to reflect on your session, what you've learned, and how you want to incorporate these insights into your day-to-day life.

1   How are you feeling? Were there any thoughts or ideas that stood out to you?

2   Were there topics that you didn't get to in this session or wish you could have kept talking about?

3   How would you like to incorporate the takeaways you noted during the session into your week?

Session 07

Use the next two pages to free write, or choose any of the
prompts below to help you get started—whatever is most helpful
for you to process and reflect in preparation for your session.

WRITING PROMPTS

- What is something you noticed more deeply recently?

- What was your favorite moment today?

- What feelings do you have that you can easily identify?
  What feelings do you have that you can't as easily name?

M | D | Y

M | D | Y

M | D | Y

M | D | Y |

M | D | Y |

M | D | Y |

Session Preparation

Take a few deep breaths. Imagine turning down the volume on all the "noise" of your day. Try to actively disconnect from any distractions, including devices, emails, or to-do lists (refer to Appendix A for Mindfulness Techniques).

When you feel ready, let's check in before your therapy session.

Pre-Session Check-In

How are you feeling right now?

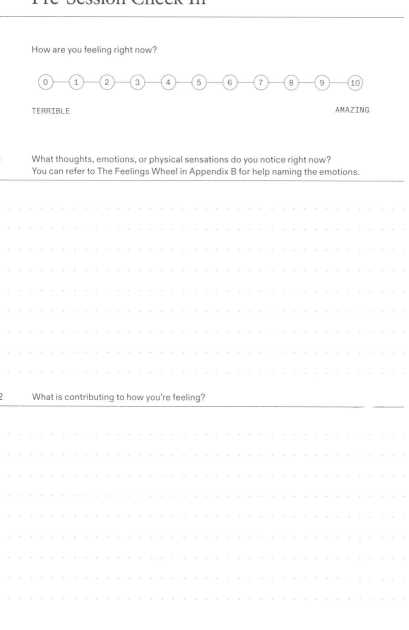

TERRIBLE   AMAZING

1   What thoughts, emotions, or physical sensations do you notice right now?
     You can refer to The Feelings Wheel in Appendix B for help naming the emotions.

2   What is contributing to how you're feeling?

Topics for This Session

What are your priorities for this session? This may include what you're currently feeling, topics from your Notes From the Week, and/or the goals you set for therapy.

1

2

3

Session Notes

Jot down helpful notes and highlights from your therapy session.

Key Takeaways

Capture the learnings, insights, and/or action items from the therapy session.

Session Reflection

Continue to reflect on your session, what you've learned, and how you want to incorporate these insights into your day-to-day life.

1   How are you feeling? Were there any thoughts or ideas that stood out to you?

2   Were there topics that you didn't get to in this session or wish you could have kept talking about?

3   How would you like to incorporate the takeaways you noted during the session into your week?

Session 08

Use the next two pages to free write, or choose any of the prompts below to help you get started—whatever is most helpful for you to process and reflect in preparation for your session.

WRITING PROMPTS

- When did you feel most challenged today?

- What is a way in which you've seen yourself grow?

- Who has offered something that felt supportive? What did they do that made you feel supported?

M | D | Y |

M | D | Y |

M | D | Y |

D	Y	

D	Y	

D	Y	

Session Preparation

Take a few deep breaths. Imagine turning down the volume on all the "noise" of your day. Try to actively disconnect from any distractions, including devices, emails, or to-do lists (refer to Appendix A for Mindfulness Techniques).

When you feel ready, let's check in before your therapy session.

Pre-Session Check-In

How are you feeling right now?

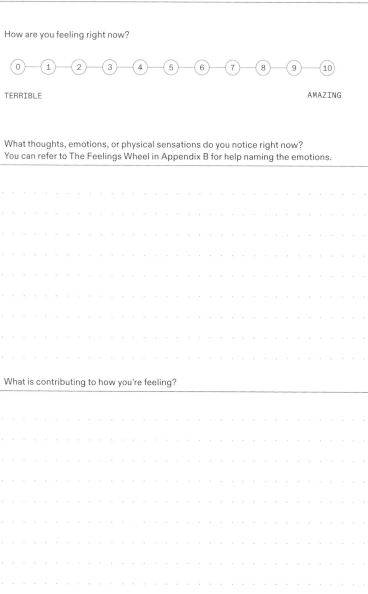

TERRIBLE   AMAZING

What thoughts, emotions, or physical sensations do you notice right now?
You can refer to The Feelings Wheel in Appendix B for help naming the emotions.

What is contributing to how you're feeling?

Topics for This Session

What are your priorities for this session? This may include what you're currently feeling, topics from your Notes From the Week, and/or the goals you set for therapy.

1

2

3

Session Notes

Jot down helpful notes and highlights from your therapy session.

Key Takeaways

Capture the learnings, insights, and/or action items from the therapy session.

Session Reflection

Continue to reflect on your session, what you've learned, and how you want to incorporate these insights into your day-to-day life.

1   How are you feeling? Were there any thoughts or ideas that stood out to you?

2   Were there topics that you didn't get to in this session or wish you could have kept talking about?

3   How would you like to incorporate the takeaways you noted during the session into your week?

Session 09

Use the next two pages to free write, or choose any of the prompts below to help you get started—whatever is most helpful for you to process and reflect in preparation for your session.

WRITING PROMPTS

- What would a trusted friend say your strengths are? Would you agree?

- How have you been affected by larger societal/political/ environmental factors recently?

- When you look in the mirror, what do you feel proud of, and what do you feel critical of?

M | D | Y |

M | D | Y |

M | D | Y |

M | D | Y |

M | D | Y |

M | D | Y |

Session Preparation

Take a few deep breaths. Imagine turning down the volume on all the "noise" of your day. Try to actively disconnect from any distractions, including devices, emails, or to-do lists (refer to Appendix A for Mindfulness Techniques).

When you feel ready, let's check in before your therapy session.

Pre-Session Check-In

How are you feeling right now?

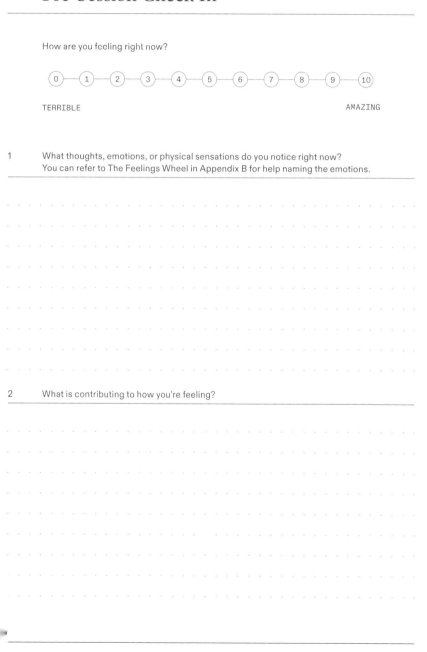

TERRIBLE   AMAZING

1   What thoughts, emotions, or physical sensations do you notice right now?
    You can refer to The Feelings Wheel in Appendix B for help naming the emotions.

2   What is contributing to how you're feeling?

Topics for This Session

What are your priorities for this session? This may include what you're currently feeling, topics from your Notes From the Week, and/or the goals you set for therapy.

1

2

3

Session Notes

Jot down helpful notes and highlights from your therapy session.

Key Takeaways

Capture the learnings, insights, and/or action items from the therapy session.

1

2

3

Session Reflection

Continue to reflect on your session, what you've learned, and how you want to incorporate these insights into your day-to-day life.

1   How are you feeling? Were there any thoughts or ideas that stood out to you?

2   Were there topics that you didn't get to in this session or wish you could have kept talking about?

3   How would you like to incorporate the takeaways you noted during the session into your week?

Session 10

Use the next two pages to free write, or choose any of the
prompts below to help you get started—whatever is most helpful
for you to process and reflect in preparation for your session.

WRITING PROMPTS

- What is a longstanding question you have about yourself
  that you'd like to think more about?

- What is something that was hard to hear initially, but
  turned out to be valuable feedback?

- What have you needed to balance this week?

M | D | Y

M | D | Y

M | D | Y

M | D | Y |

M | D | Y |

| D | Y |

Session Preparation

Take a few deep breaths. Imagine turning down the volume on all the "noise" of your day. Try to actively disconnect from any distractions, including devices, emails, or to-do lists (refer to Appendix A for Mindfulness Techniques).

When you feel ready, let's check in before your therapy session.

Pre-Session Check-In

How are you feeling right now?

(0) — (1) — (2) — (3) — (4) — (5) — (6) — (7) — (8) — (9) — (10)

TERRIBLE   AMAZING

1   What thoughts, emotions, or physical sensations do you notice right now?
     You can refer to The Feelings Wheel in Appendix B for help naming the emotions.

2   What is contributing to how you're feeling?

Topics for This Session

What are your priorities for this session? This may include what you're currently feeling,
topics from your Notes From the Week, and/or the goals you set for therapy.

1

2

3

Session Notes

Jot down helpful notes and highlights from your therapy session.

Key Takeaways

Capture the learnings, insights, and/or action items from the therapy session.

Session Reflection

Continue to reflect on your session, what you've learned, and how you want to incorporate these insights into your day-to-day life.

1   How are you feeling? Were there any thoughts or ideas that stood out to you?

2   Were there topics that you didn't get to in this session or wish you could have kept
         talking about?

3   How would you like to incorporate the takeaways you noted during the session
         into your week?

Goal Check-In

Now that you've been working in therapy for a while, it's a good time to check in. Reflect on the goal you set at the beginning of this journal. Then, check in on your relationship with your therapist.

1   What changes (to your behavior, habits, thought patterns, etc.) have you
     noticed since starting therapy? Have you made progress towards your goal?

2   During the course of therapy, what topics outside your goal have come up?
     Are they more important or pressing to address?

3   Are there changes that need to be made to your therapy goal? If so, write
     down your updated goal here:

Therapist Check-In

A strong therapeutic alliance is a key ingredient for successful therapy outcomes.[8] Research shows that this relationship comes from having a trusting bond with the clinician and being in agreement on your goals.[9] Let's check in on your relationship with your therapist.

1   What has stood out to you in your interactions together?

2   Do you think you're getting what you wanted out of therapy? What would you change, if anything, about your therapy and your relationship with your therapist?

NEXT STEPS

Based on your responses, it may be helpful to discuss how
things are going with your therapist. Here are some guidelines for how to navigate that conversation:

- If your goal has changed or a key component of your
  therapy relationship is missing, communicate that to your
  therapist so they can be more effective in helping you.
  If you feel poorly about how therapy is going, they likely
  feel it, too.

- If you and your therapist have been doing good work
  together, it can be helpful to share what has made this a
  positive experience. This is an opportunity to foster depth
  and openness within the relationship.

- If you need help deciding whether it's time to switch
  therapists, see Appendix D for more guidance.

Session 11

Use the next two pages to free write, or choose any of the prompts below to help you get started—whatever is most helpful for you to process and reflect in preparation for your session.

WRITING PROMPTS

- Have your actions been influenced by self-criticism or self-judgment recently? If so, how?

- When you reflect on your day, what do you think your therapist would commend you for?

- What were some feelings you recognized and acknowledged today?

M | D | Y |

M | D | Y |

M | D | Y |

M	D	Y	

	D	Y	

	D	Y	

Session Preparation

Take a few deep breaths. Imagine turning down the volume on all the "noise" of your day. Try to actively disconnect from any distractions, including devices, emails, or to-do lists (refer to Appendix A for Mindfulness Techniques).

When you feel ready, let's check in before your therapy session.

Pre-Session Check-In

How are you feeling right now?

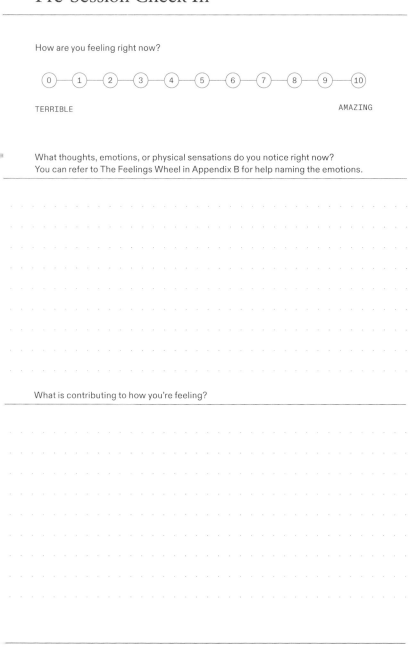

(0)—(1)—(2)—(3)—(4)—(5)—(6)—(7)—(8)—(9)—(10)

TERRIBLE   AMAZING

What thoughts, emotions, or physical sensations do you notice right now?
You can refer to The Feelings Wheel in Appendix B for help naming the emotions.

What is contributing to how you're feeling?

Topics for This Session

What are your priorities for this session? This may include what you're currently feeling,
topics from your Notes From the Week, and/or the goals you set for therapy.

1

2

3

Session Notes

Jot down helpful notes and highlights from your therapy session.

Key Takeaways

Capture the learnings, insights, and/or action items from the therapy session.

1

2

3

Session Reflection

Continue to reflect on your session, what you've learned, and how you want to incorporate these insights into your day-to-day life.

1   How are you feeling? Were there any thoughts or ideas that stood out to you?

2   Were there topics that you didn't get to in this session or wish you could have kept talking about?

3   How would you like to incorporate the takeaways you noted during the session into your week?

Session 12

Use the next two pages to free write, or choose any of the prompts below to help you get started—whatever is most helpful for you to process and reflect in preparation for your session.

WRITING PROMPTS

- What kind of support would you like to receive right now?

- What does self-compassion look like for you right now?

- What do you want to lean into, and what do you want to pull back from?

M | D | Y |

M | D | Y |

M | D | Y |

M | D | Y |

M | D | Y |

M | D | Y |

Session Preparation

Take a few deep breaths. Imagine turning down the volume on all the "noise" of your day. Try to actively disconnect from any distractions, including devices, emails, or to-do lists (refer to Appendix A for Mindfulness Techniques).

When you feel ready, let's check in before your therapy session.

Pre-Session Check-In

How are you feeling right now?

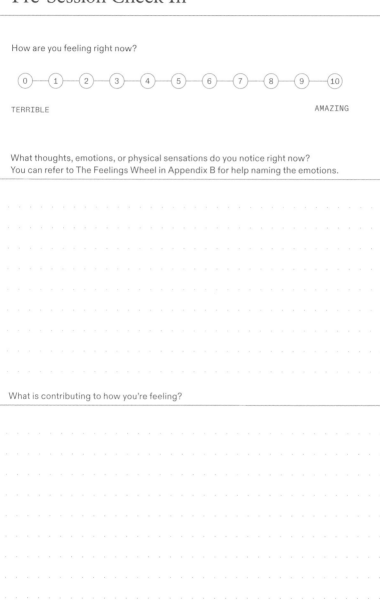

(0)—(1)—(2)—(3)—(4)—(5)—(6)—(7)—(8)—(9)—(10)

TERRIBLE   AMAZING

What thoughts, emotions, or physical sensations do you notice right now?
You can refer to The Feelings Wheel in Appendix B for help naming the emotions.

What is contributing to how you're feeling?

Topics for This Session

What are your priorities for this session? This may include what you're currently feeling, topics from your Notes From the Week, and/or the goals you set for therapy.

1

2

3

Session Notes

Jot down helpful notes and highlights from your therapy session.

Key Takeaways

Capture the learnings, insights, and/or action items from the therapy session.

Session Reflection

Continue to reflect on your session, what you've learned, and how you want to incorporate these insights into your day-to-day life.

1   How are you feeling? Were there any thoughts or ideas that stood out to you?

2   Were there topics that you didn't get to in this session or wish you could have kept talking about?

3   How would you like to incorporate the takeaways you noted during the session into your week?

Session 13

Use the next two pages to free write, or choose any of the prompts below to help you get started—whatever is most helpful for you to process and reflect in preparation for your session.

WRITING PROMPTS

- How did you cope today (with stress, intense emotions, etc.)?

- What are your current physical, mental, emotional, and social needs?

- What did you do recently to build, strengthen, or maintain a relationship?

M | D | Y |

M | D | Y |

M | D | Y |

M | D | Y |

M | D | Y |

M | D | Y |

Session Preparation

Take a few deep breaths. Imagine turning down the volume on all the "noise" of your day. Try to actively disconnect from any distractions, including devices, emails, or to-do lists (refer to Appendix A for Mindfulness Techniques).

When you feel ready, let's check in before your therapy session.

Pre-Session Check-In

How are you feeling right now?

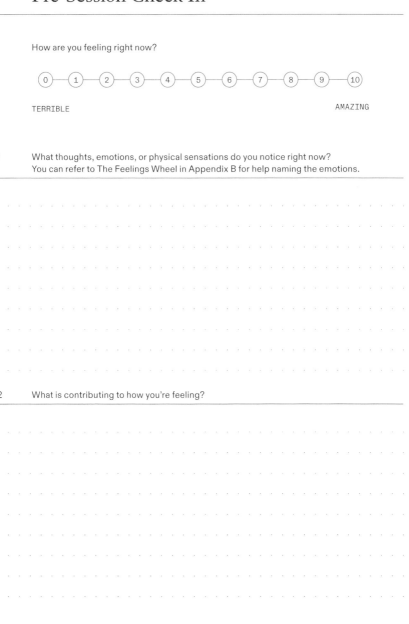

TERRIBLE   AMAZING

1   What thoughts, emotions, or physical sensations do you notice right now?
You can refer to The Feelings Wheel in Appendix B for help naming the emotions.

2   What is contributing to how you're feeling?

Topics for This Session

What are your priorities for this session? This may include what you're currently feeling, topics from your Notes From the Week, and/or the goals you set for therapy.

1

2

3

Session Notes

Jot down helpful notes and highlights from your therapy session.

Key Takeaways

Capture the learnings, insights, and/or action items from the therapy session.

Session Reflection

Continue to reflect on your session, what you've learned, and how you want to incorporate these insights into your day-to-day life.

1   How are you feeling? Were there any thoughts or ideas that stood out to you?

2   Were there topics that you didn't get to in this session or wish you could have kept talking about?

3   How would you like to incorporate the takeaways you noted during the session into your week?

Session 14

Use the next two pages to free write, or choose any of the prompts below to help you get started—whatever is most helpful for you to process and reflect in preparation for your session.

WRITING PROMPTS

- What barriers to your therapy work have you noticed recently?

- What did you do to be kind to yourself today?

- What are you looking forward to?

M | D | Y |

M | D | Y |

M | D | Y |

M | D | Y

M | D | Y

M | D | Y

Session Preparation

Take a few deep breaths. Imagine turning down the volume on all the "noise" of your day. Try to actively disconnect from any distractions, including devices, emails, or to-do lists (refer to Appendix A for Mindfulness Techniques).

When you feel ready, let's check in before your therapy session.

Pre-Session Check-In

How are you feeling right now?

(0)—(1)—(2)—(3)—(4)—(5)—(6)—(7)—(8)—(9)—(10)

TERRIBLE   AMAZING

1   What thoughts, emotions, or physical sensations do you notice right now?
     You can refer to The Feelings Wheel in Appendix B for help naming the emotions.

2   What is contributing to how you're feeling?

Topics for This Session

What are your priorities for this session? This may include what you're currently feeling, topics from your Notes From the Week, and/or the goals you set for therapy.

1

2

3

Session Notes

Jot down helpful notes and highlights from your therapy session.

Key Takeaways

Capture the learnings, insights, and/or action items from the therapy session.

Session Reflection

Continue to reflect on your session, what you've learned, and how you want to incorporate these insights into your day-to-day life.

1   How are you feeling? Were there any thoughts or ideas that stood out to you?

2   Were there topics that you didn't get to in this session or wish you could have kept talking about?

3   How would you like to incorporate the takeaways you noted during the session into your week?

Session 15

Use the next two pages to free write, or choose any of the prompts below to help you get started—whatever is most helpful for you to process and reflect in preparation for your session.

WRITING PROMPTS

- What are some activities you'd like to try or to do more often?

- When did you most recently feel empowered?

- How would you support a friend who experienced your challenges this week?

M | D | Y

M | D | Y

M | D | Y

M | D | Y |

M | D | Y |

M | D | Y |

Session Preparation

Take a few deep breaths. Imagine turning down the volume on all the "noise" of your day. Try to actively disconnect from any distractions, including devices, emails, or to-do lists (refer to Appendix A for Mindfulness Techniques).

When you feel ready, let's check in before your therapy session.

Pre-Session Check-In

How are you feeling right now?

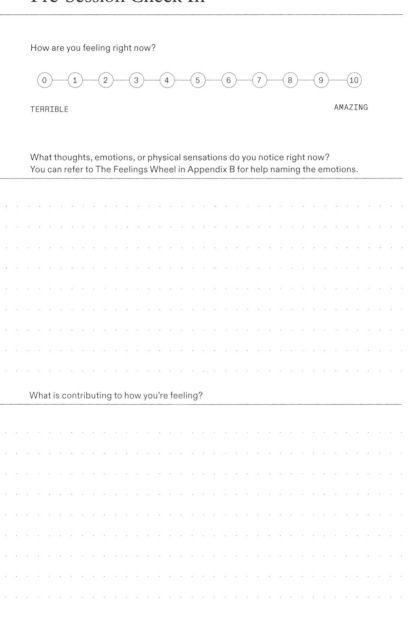

(0) — (1) — (2) — (3) — (4) — (5) — (6) — (7) — (8) — (9) — (10)

TERRIBLE   AMAZING

1   What thoughts, emotions, or physical sensations do you notice right now?
        You can refer to The Feelings Wheel in Appendix B for help naming the emotions.

2   What is contributing to how you're feeling?

Topics for This Session

What are your priorities for this session? This may include what you're currently feeling,
topics from your Notes From the Week, and/or the goals you set for therapy.

1

2

3

Session Notes

Jot down helpful notes and highlights from your therapy session.

Key Takeaways

Capture the learnings, insights, and/or action items from the therapy session.

Session Reflection

Continue to reflect on your session, what you've learned, and how you want to incorporate these insights into your day-to-day life.

1   How are you feeling? Were there any thoughts or ideas that stood out to you?

2   Were there topics that you didn't get to in this session or wish you could have kept talking about?

3   How would you like to incorporate the takeaways you noted during the session into your week?

Session 16

Use the next two pages to free write, or choose any of the prompts below to help you get started—whatever is most helpful for you to process and reflect in preparation for your session.

WRITING PROMPTS

- What excites you?

- How did you manage intense feelings recently?
  How effective was it?

- What are things that you rarely, if ever, worry about?

M | D | Y

M | D | Y

M | D | Y

M | D | Y |

M | D | Y |

M | D | Y |

Session Preparation

Take a few deep breaths. Imagine turning down the volume on all the "noise" of your day. Try to actively disconnect from any distractions, including devices, emails, or to-do lists (refer to Appendix A for Mindfulness Techniques).

When you feel ready, let's check in before your therapy session.

Pre-Session Check-In

How are you feeling right now?

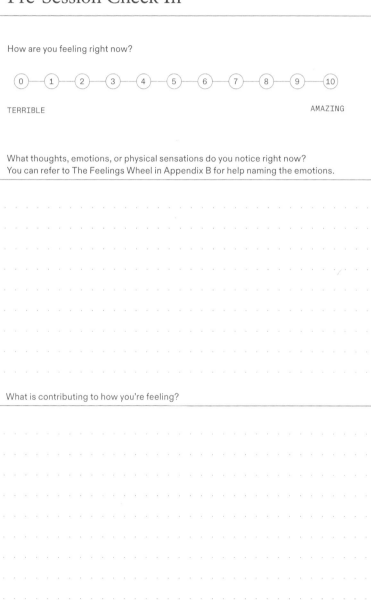

TERRIBLE   AMAZING

1   What thoughts, emotions, or physical sensations do you notice right now?
      You can refer to The Feelings Wheel in Appendix B for help naming the emotions.

2   What is contributing to how you're feeling?

Topics for This Session

What are your priorities for this session? This may include what you're currently feeling, topics from your Notes From the Week, and/or the goals you set for therapy.

1

2

3

Session Notes

Jot down helpful notes and highlights from your therapy session.

Key Takeaways

Capture the learnings, insights, and/or action items from the therapy session.

Session Reflection

Continue to reflect on your session, what you've learned, and how you want to incorporate these insights into your day-to-day life.

1   How are you feeling? Were there any thoughts or ideas that stood out to you?

2   Were there topics that you didn't get to in this session or wish you could have kept talking about?

3   How would you like to incorporate the takeaways you noted during the session into your week?

Session 17

Use the next two pages to free write, or choose any of the prompts below to help you get started—whatever is most helpful for you to process and reflect in preparation for your session.

WRITING PROMPTS

- What is something you've done to take care of yourself today?

- Who made the biggest impact on you today? Why?

- What effect has your home or environment had on you recently?

M | D | Y |

M | D | Y |

M | D | Y |

	D	Y

	D	Y

	D	Y

Session Preparation

Take a few deep breaths. Imagine turning down the volume on all the "noise" of your day. Try to actively disconnect from any distractions, including devices, emails, or to-do lists (refer to Appendix A for Mindfulness Techniques).

When you feel ready, let's check in before your therapy session.

Pre-Session Check-In

How are you feeling right now?

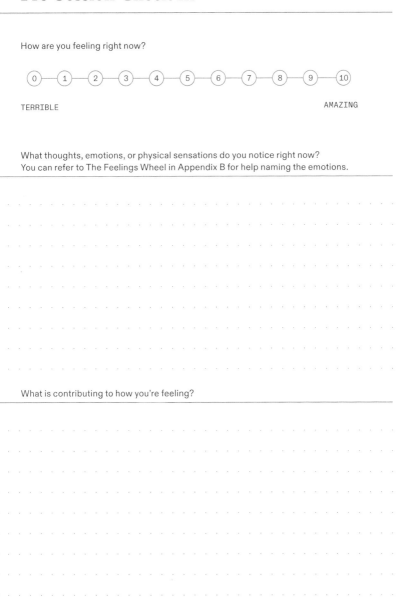

⓪—①—②—③—④—⑤—⑥—⑦—⑧—⑨—⑩

TERRIBLE   AMAZING

What thoughts, emotions, or physical sensations do you notice right now?
You can refer to The Feelings Wheel in Appendix B for help naming the emotions.

What is contributing to how you're feeling?

Topics for This Session

What are your priorities for this session? This may include what you're currently feeling, topics from your Notes From the Week, and/or the goals you set for therapy.

1

2

3

Session Notes

Jot down helpful notes and highlights from your therapy session.

Key Takeaways

Capture the learnings, insights, and/or action items from the therapy session.

Session Reflection

Continue to reflect on your session, what you've learned, and how you want to incorporate these insights into your day-to-day life.

1   How are you feeling? Were there any thoughts or ideas that stood out to you?

2   Were there topics that you didn't get to in this session or wish you could have kept talking about?

3   How would you like to incorporate the takeaways you noted during the session into your week?

Session 18

Use the next two pages to free write, or choose any of the prompts below to help you get started—whatever is most helpful for you to process and reflect in preparation for your session.

WRITING PROMPTS

- What do you think others admire about you?

- What are your go-to activities to unwind and recharge?

- How has the past shown up and impacted you recently?

M | D | Y |

M | D | Y |

M | D | Y |

M | D | Y |

M | D | Y |

M | D | Y |

Session Preparation

Take a few deep breaths. Imagine turning down the volume on all the "noise" of your day. Try to actively disconnect from any distractions, including devices, emails, or to-do lists (refer to Appendix A for Mindfulness Techniques).

When you feel ready, let's check in before your therapy session.

Pre-Session Check-In

How are you feeling right now?

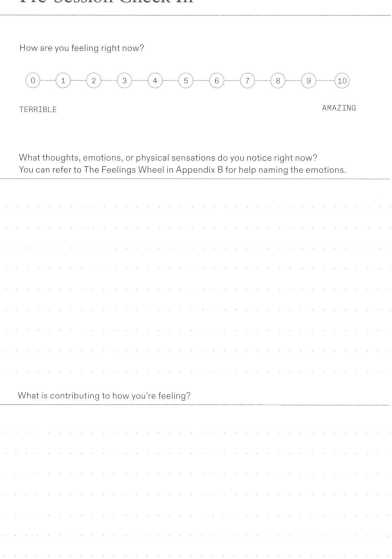

TERRIBLE   AMAZING

1   What thoughts, emotions, or physical sensations do you notice right now?
    You can refer to The Feelings Wheel in Appendix B for help naming the emotions.

2   What is contributing to how you're feeling?

Topics for This Session

What are your priorities for this session? This may include what you're currently feeling, topics from your Notes From the Week, and/or the goals you set for therapy.

1

2

3

Session Notes

Jot down helpful notes and highlights from your therapy session.

Key Takeaways

Capture the learnings, insights, and/or action items from the therapy session.

1

2

3

Session Reflection

Continue to reflect on your session, what you've learned, and how you want to incorporate these insights into your day-to-day life.

1   How are you feeling? Were there any thoughts or ideas that stood out to you?

2   Were there topics that you didn't get to in this session or wish you could have kept talking about?

3   How would you like to incorporate the takeaways you noted during the session into your week?

Session 19

Use the next two pages to free write, or choose any of the prompts below to help you get started—whatever is most helpful for you to process and reflect in preparation for your session.

WRITING PROMPTS

•   What is something you experienced that brought you joy?

•   What do you feel proud of?

•   How has your breath felt today? How does your body feel?

M | D | Y |

M | D | Y |

M | D | Y |

M | D | Y

M | D | Y

M | D | Y

Session Preparation

Take a few deep breaths. Imagine turning down the volume on all the "noise" of your day. Try to actively disconnect from any distractions, including devices, emails, or to-do lists (refer to Appendix A for Mindfulness Techniques).

When you feel ready, let's check in before your therapy session.

Pre-Session Check-In

How are you feeling right now?

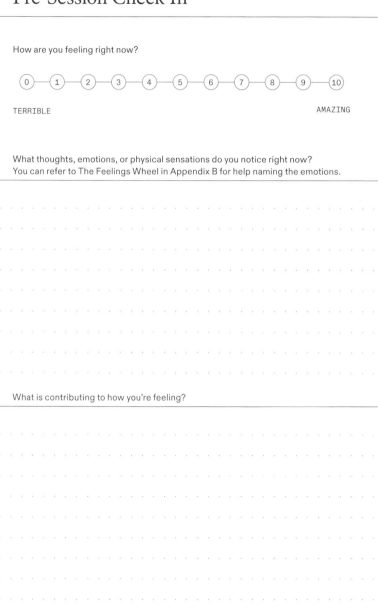

(0)—(1)—(2)—(3)—(4)—(5)—(6)—(7)—(8)—(9)—(10)

TERRIBLE   AMAZING

1   What thoughts, emotions, or physical sensations do you notice right now?
        You can refer to The Feelings Wheel in Appendix B for help naming the emotions.

2   What is contributing to how you're feeling?

Topics for This Session

What are your priorities for this session? This may include what you're currently feeling, topics from your Notes From the Week, and/or the goals you set for therapy.

1

2

3

Session Notes

Jot down helpful notes and highlights from your therapy session.

Key Takeaways

Capture the learnings, insights, and/or action items from the therapy session.

1

2

3

Session Reflection

Continue to reflect on your session, what you've learned, and how you want to incorporate these insights into your day-to-day life.

1   How are you feeling? Were there any thoughts or ideas that stood out to you?

2   Were there topics that you didn't get to in this session or wish you could have kept talking about?

3   How would you like to incorporate the takeaways you noted during the session into your week?

Session 20

Use the next two pages to free write, or choose any of the prompts below to help you get started—whatever is most helpful for you to process and reflect in preparation for your session.

WRITING PROMPTS

- What has the tone of your self-talk been lately?

- What do you most feel like doing right now?

- What kind of movement or activity has felt joyful or empowering recently?

M | D | Y |

M | D | Y |

M | D | Y |

M | D | Y |

M | D | Y |

M | D | Y |

Session Preparation

Take a few deep breaths. Imagine turning down the volume on all the "noise" of your day. Try to actively disconnect from any distractions, including devices, emails, or to-do lists (refer to Appendix A for Mindfulness Techniques).

When you feel ready, let's check in before your therapy session.

Pre-Session Check-In

How are you feeling right now?

(0)—(1)—(2)—(3)—(4)—(5)—(6)—(7)—(8)—(9)—(10)

TERRIBLE   AMAZING

1   What thoughts, emotions, or physical sensations do you notice right now?
     You can refer to The Feelings Wheel in Appendix B for help naming the emotions.

2   What is contributing to how you're feeling?

Topics for This Session

What are your priorities for this session? This may include what you're currently feeling, topics from your Notes From the Week, and/or the goals you set for therapy.

1

2

3

Session Notes

Jot down helpful notes and highlights from your therapy session.

Key Takeaways

Capture the learnings, insights, and/or action items from the therapy session.

1

2

3

Session Reflection

Continue to reflect on your session, what you've learned, and how you want to incorporate these insights into your day-to-day life.

1   How are you feeling? Were there any thoughts or ideas that stood out to you?

2   Were there topics that you didn't get to in this session or wish you could have kept talking about?

3   How would you like to incorporate the takeaways you noted during the session into your week?

Goal Check-In

Now that you've been working in therapy for a while, it's a good time to check in. Reflect on the goal you set at the beginning of this journal. Then, check in on your relationship with your therapist.

1   What changes (to your behavior, habits, thought patterns, etc.) have you
        noticed since starting therapy? Have you made progress towards your goal?

2   During the course of therapy, what topics outside your goal have come up?
        Are they more important or pressing to address?

3   Are there changes that need to be made to your therapy goal? If so, write
        down your updated goal here:

Therapist Check-In

Reflect on your relationship with your therapist. Consider your sense of trust with them, as well as the effectiveness of your work together.

1   What has stood out to you in your interactions together?

2   Do you think you're getting what you wanted out of therapy? What would you change, if anything, about your therapy and your relationship with your therapist?

NEXT STEPS

Based on your responses, it may be helpful to discuss how things are going with your therapist. Here are some guidelines for how to navigate that conversation:

- If your goal has changed or a key component of your therapy relationship is missing, communicate that to your therapist so they can be more effective in helping you. If you feel poorly about how therapy is going, they likely feel it, too.

- If you and your therapist have been doing good work together, it can be helpful to share what has made this a positive experience. This is an opportunity to foster depth and openness within the relationship.

- If you need help deciding whether it's time to switch therapists, see Appendix D for more guidance.

A   Mindfulness Techniques

We understand that it can be difficult to transition into or out of a therapy mindset, and that intense feelings can come up that you may need help moving through.

Here are a few different ways to reorient to yourself and your surroundings:

SQUARE BREATHING

Trace your finger along the sides of the square slowly, counting to four or five on each side. Start with a deep inhale, hold that breath, then release a slow exhale. Hold at the bottom of the breath.

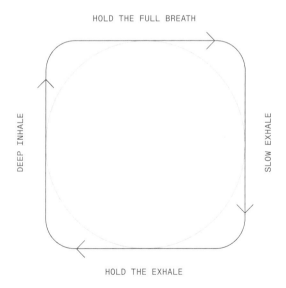

GROUNDING THROUGH SENSES

Bring your full attention to something readily accessible, such as a small object nearby, music, food or drink, or something you're wearing. Consider some of the following:

What can you notice using your:

Sight

What does it look like? What textures does it have? What lines or shapes are involved? What color is it? How opaque or transparent is it?

Touch

What does it feel like? What temperature is it? Is it smooth or rough? How soft or firm? How might it feel using your fingertips or nails versus your palm? What ridges or tactile contrast is there?

Smell or taste

How would this be described in a book? What are your first impressions, and what shows up when you continue to focus on it? Would you consider it savory or sweet; floral or woodsy; airy or complex?

Hearing

What sounds do you hear? How near or far are they? What sort of pitch and tone are they? Are they consistent or intermittent? What are other, softer sounds you can notice as well?

BRIEF PROGRESSIVE MUSCLE RELAXATION

This exercise asks you to tense up various muscle groups as tightly as you can for about five seconds at a time, then fully release. Notice the difference in tension and relaxation.

Starting from the bottom of the body:

Legs like a ballerina

Point your toes as hard as you can, and tighten your calves, thighs, and buttocks. Hold it as tightly as possible for five slow counts, before you fully release.

Back like a bow

Pull your shoulders back and gently arch your back until it feels tight. Hold the tension and muscles as tightly as possible for five counts. Then, release it fully.

Arms like a bodybuilder

With your arms up and fists curled, tense your biceps, forearms, and stomach as much as you can. Hold the tension for five seconds, then let it go.

Face like a walnut

Clench your jaw, purse your lips, scrunch your nose, and squeeze your eyes closed for five seconds. Hold this as tightly as you can. Then, relax your face.

DIAPHRAGMATIC BREATHING (BELLY BREATHS)

This is a form of breathing in which you focus on inhaling down into your stomach instead of shallowly into your lungs. It is often helpful to place one hand on the belly, or right above the beltline, and the other hand on your chest.

Imagine a balloon in your stomach.

- As you inhale, focus on filling up this balloon, pushing your lower hand out. Do your best to keep your upper hand still.

- As you exhale, focus on deflating this balloon in your stomach.

While this focus on your breath can make it feel tight or ragged initially, over time it mimics the gentle deep breathing during sleep, and will help your body relax.

PAIRED CUE BODY SCAN

In this exercise, you'll observe your body and notice tension within it, then utilize your breath to help release the tension. Select a "cue" word, such as "release", "relax", "calm" or "unwind". Over time, you will start to pair the cue word with the feeling of relaxing your body, and the word itself can help you de-stress.

- Starting from your toes and legs, notice if there is any tension in these parts of the body. If there is, take a deep breath in, and on the exhale, focus on releasing whatever muscles are being held taut. As you do so, say your cue word to yourself. For example, if I noticed I was keeping myself on my toes, with my calves tight, I would take a deep breath, then relax my calves as I say "release" to myself.

- Move up the body scan to your stomach, again allowing it to relax as you exhale and say your cue word.

- Then, check in with your neck, arms, and hands, taking a deep breath in so that you can release your breath at the same time as you release the tension.

- Moving up to your jaw, forehead, and face, check for tension and take a moment to release it with your breath and your cue word together.

VISUALIZATION

It can be helpful to visualize a calming scene to help your mind and body unwind. What feels calming is unique to each person, but is often informed by previous enjoyable and relaxing experiences. While people may often choose beach or wooded scenes, some may also choose something a little closer to home, such as the first moment of lying down in bed, or a particularly relaxing moment with a pet. Some create their own based on their imagination or other images they've seen.

Whatever the image, bring it to mind vividly so that you can truly see yourself there and be transported.

- Consider what small details might be in the scene: what you can see, feel on your body, hear, and smell.

- Include enough detail that an artist could draw the vignette, so you can remember and come back to this place in your mind.

- Give yourself several minutes to explore and indulge in this scene and the relaxing feeling associated with it.

COUNTED BREATHS

This exercise will regulate your breath to slow your heart rate.

Inhale deeply for a slow count of four, and exhale fully for a slow count of five. Continue to inhale, then exhale for one more count.

As you feel yourself connecting to your breath, you can increase how long you inhale and exhale for, such as inhaling for a count of six, then exhaling for a count of seven.

B   The Feelings Wheel

This graphic is a flexible tool to help you identify your feelings.

Some people like to start from the inner rings of the circle and work their way out to identify greater nuance to their feelings. Others like to scan the entire circle freely to see what words jump out at them. Do what works for you.

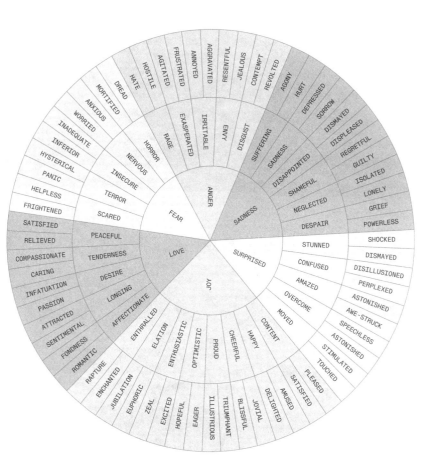

C   Fundamentals of Self-Care

You may be seeking therapy because other ways you've tried to make change haven't worked. But, we also don't want to understate the value of tending to your basic needs.

Below, you'll find a list of fundamental self-care practices to consider and implement into your life. When well-addressed, they can improve your mood, coping ability, and overall health.[10] Taking care of these foundational elements can be an immensely helpful partner to your therapeutic work.

NUTRITION

Maintaining your body's nutritional needs is essential for regulating your mood. Your ability to think, communicate effectively, and manage your emotions is directly impacted by food. Notice how and when your body responds to certain foods, and if there are enhancements to your mood and energy levels.

Example: Try to feed yourself throughout the day (three or more mealtimes is a good reference point), doing your best to include a variety of food groups.

EXERCISE

Movement relieves endorphins, which in turn relieve stress. Physical activity can also help give your body space to move through feelings, your mind to process thoughts, and your self-esteem a sense of accomplishment.

Example: Try stretching while watching TV, having a mini-dance party, or walking around the block when you want to clear your head.

SUBSTANCE USE

Caffeine, alcohol, cannabis, and other substances can disrupt your ability to control your emotions and thoughts. Be aware of excessive or unhelpful use.

Example: A way to limit substances is to buy less so that there's less on hand, and to put it in inconvenient places (e.g. above the fridge or in the back of a closet) to make it harder to access.

PHYSICAL HEALTH

Illnesses, chronic issues including stress, and hormonal imbalances can take a toll on your mental health and sometimes mimic the symptoms of certain disorders.

Example: Make regular check-ups a priority, and be sure to speak to your doctor about any mental health symptoms.

SLEEP

Sufficient quantity (7-9 hours for most people) and quality of sleep are both important. Studies continue to show how sufficient sleep improves the brain's ability to regulate emotions and keeps mood and anxiety levels from worsening.[11]

Example: Try to use your bed only for sleep and keep a regular bedtime. Designate a different area for TV, work, and other "daytime" activities.

MINDFULNESS

Over the past decade, studies have shown that mindfulness practices may physically increase the size of brain regions associated with regulating emotion.[12] The practice of being non-judgmentally aware of the present moment can help with building insight, feeling calmer, and having the space to react more effectively to a situation.

Example: Take a moment to name five things you see, four things you touch, three sounds, two smells, and one taste. Finish by taking one really deep breath. You can reference more techniques in Appendix A.

SOCIAL CONNECTION

Quality social relationships improve lifespan and reduce risk for heart disease, among many other physical and mental health benefits.[13] Trusted relationships can provide an outlet for venting, different perspectives, and understanding.

Example: Consider who has been helpful and safe for you and what it was that they did. It may be worth asking directly for that kind of support in the future, or expressing gratitude for it.

D   How Do I Know if My Therapist is a Good Fit?

Your therapist is your co-pilot and collaborator throughout your therapy journey, and an essential part of your progress.

For many, it may have been so difficult to navigate their health insurance or find a therapist that they think, "We'll just make it work!" or "Something is better than nothing." However, it's important for the therapy relationship and your treatment that you feel comfortable with your therapist and reasonably confident that the treatment you're undergoing together will be beneficial.

We've summarized a few considerations to help you determine whether or not a therapist is a good fit. Our questions here are not exhaustive, and the determination of fit is ultimately up to you.

Here are some things to consider:

- Do they seem to understand you?

- Do they appear to respect you and what you're saying?

- If you clarify or disagree with something they've said, are they open to hearing and incorporating it?

- Do you believe that they have the right expertise and experience to help you?

- Do the things they suggest help you with your therapy goals?

- Do you feel there is trust with this therapist?

The hope is that, over the course of a few sessions, your answer to most of these questions is "yes." If you find that some of these are more consistently a "no," you should first consider sharing your feedback with the therapist. As difficult or potentially awkward as this conversation can be, giving this feedback can lead to a new, deeper understanding of both parties and result in a much stronger therapeutic relationship.

It gives your therapist more insight into how your mind works and shows that you trust them to adjust the approach according to your needs. Chances are, your therapist will appreciate this feedback.

On the other hand, if you don't believe that the two of you can work well together, then you'll want to look at ending this therapy relationship. This is especially true if you cannot assume good intentions and don't believe that the therapy can be adjusted. Ideally, you would still tell the therapist why you are ending the relationship: that you aren't getting what you would like out of therapy, that there seems to be a mismatch in communication, or that you may be needing a different style or approach. With this feedback, the therapist may also be able to connect you to someone who may be a better fit, and you can reflect together on what could have been improved.

Sometimes therapy can be emotionally challenging and you may feel reflexively hurt or upset by something a therapist says. This doesn't necessarily mean your therapist did anything wrong and could in fact be a therapeutic moment of being honest about your reaction. However, there are some situations in which ending the relationship abruptly is in your best interest. If the therapist seems to be actively doing harm (by belittling you, saying disrespectful or hurtful things, or suggesting things that are clearly ill-advised), then you should prioritize your emotional safety and end the relationship immediately. You also have the option of filing a complaint with the state or province licensing board if you believe others may also be harmed by this clinician.

E   Therapist FAQ

Q: *I've talked about this issue with friends and others already.*

A: *What more will the therapist add?*

Friends and family are great sources of support and can provide alternative perspectives. Through skills and training, therapists bring an unbiased outside perspective and a nonjudgmental space in which to reflect and explore paths you may not have known existed.

Q: *Can't a therapist just fix my problems?*

A: There can be moments of insight that feel like a therapist has made some sort of magic happen. However, therapy is a highly active process. Change is limited if the client is not ready or willing to engage in the therapeutic process. Therapists rely on you to bring your knowledge of yourself, share your inner experiences, and be open to new ideas or perspectives.

Q: *Therapy is so expensive. What are my options?*

A: Therapy can, unfortunately, be very expensive. Rates are typically informed by cost of living, business overhead, and maintaining licensure. If available to you, utilize your health insurance and Employee Assistance Program. Understand what your mental health options and insurance benefits are, including your employer-covered yearly sessions, deductible (how much you're responsible for before insurance starts paying), your copay or co-insurance (the fixed amount or percentage of the cost you'll be responsible for), and your out-of-pocket maximum (the maximum you'd pay in a year before insurance covers everything). Check this for both in-network and out-of-network providers, and see what is within your budget.

     If you don't have insurance, or your health insurance costs are too high, then ask providers if they have sliding scale options (rates that are dependent on income or financial need). Therapists recognize that many people are in this situation and do their best to be respectful of varying financial situations. You can also look into options such as community mental health clinics, graduate psychology training clinics, and sources like Open Path, a network of therapists which offers sessions at a reduced rate.

     If this all sounds overwhelming (it would be understandable!), lean on your support network to help you get the care you need. If picking up the phone seems hard, your loved ones can call therapists or look up directories via affordable networks for you.

     These are options for individual therapy. If that isn't accessible, another option is group therapy. As the name implies, group therapy occurs with many clients at once, with one or two providers leading the session. They take a variety of forms, from structured groups to focus on learning skills, to open-ended groups to process and build insight, to even Dungeons and Dragons groups to help social anxiety and interpersonal issues! These tend to be cheaper per session and can be a great way to have support and shared experiences with others who struggle with similar issues.

It is also possible to invest in yourself through self-help methods. Of course, Therapy Notebooks is a great resource for working through some things yourself, as are other self-help workbooks. If there is a specific topic you are looking for, you can also find therapists who specialize in this issue and reach out to them to ask about self-help resources. Even if they aren't accepting new clients, they may have some books, websites, podcasts, or other resources that they regularly refer their clients to.

Q: *What's the difference between therapy and psychiatry?*

A: There is a multitude of mental health services and resources available, and they often have lots of acronyms or similar-sounding names, which only makes it more confusing and difficult to identify what might actually help you.

Therapy consists of services to help people with mental health struggles, and can take the form of individual meetings, meetings with family or significant others, or group meetings with multiple people with similar experiences. It is typically with licensed providers who are psychologists (PhD or PsyD), mental health counselors (LMHC), professional clinical counselors (LPCC), clinical social workers (LCSW), or marriage and family therapists (LMFT). All of these people serve as therapists and have received the required graduate training to do so. While there are some differences in training between the LMHC, LPCC, LCSW, and LMFT licenses, they are all equipped to provide psychotherapy, and oftentimes differ simply based on a state's nomenclature.

Medication management within mental health is a service to help people with psychotropic medication, or medications that manage mood and psychological conditions. People who can help with this are doctors such as primary care physicians or general practitioners (MD), psychiatrists (MD), psychiatric nurse practitioners (ARNP or PMHNP), or family nurse practitioners (FNP). Typically, conditions other than anxiety and depression are better handled by more specialized providers, such as psychiatrists and psychiatric nurse practitioners who have received more training on various medications, side effects, and interactions.

Q: *Will my therapist recommend medication?*

A: Not necessarily. Medication is another resource that can be very helpful for managing symptoms or mood. When symptoms interfere with your life, your therapist may suggest medication. This often makes therapy easier to engage in. This way of managing symptoms through medication while working to make broader changes through therapy has been supported in the literature as more effective than either alone. Medication is also recommended when it is the most evidence-based treatment for managing a condition, such as bipolar disorder or ADHD.

Q: *How long can I expect to be in therapy?*

A: This varies a lot from person to person. Unless you're in a highly structured therapy (DBT skills group, for example), the course of therapy is entirely dependent on the progress you make and what you and your provider feel is appropriate.

While most people will meet weekly, some will have sessions every other week or twice a week. Once a week tends to be the default because it's enough time for you to try new things and reflect. If you're having a hard time coming up with things to talk about after a week, or if you've been anxiously awaiting the next session, consider discussing this with your therapist to determine the root cause and if you need to change your session frequency.

Q: *Is it okay to stop going to therapy, and then start again later?*

A: Yes, absolutely. There are lots of reasons why someone may need to or choose to end treatment, including resolution of the initial issue, poor fit or lack of progress, or logistical issues. It's normal to feel sad or ambivalent about saying goodbye to your therapist. If you can, allow time to process the end of this relationship and chapter.

It's also normal to restart therapy in the future, with either the same or a new therapist, if you notice yourself struggling or wanting more support. These issues may be things you've talked about and worked on previously, or a new issue. Know that it's okay to ask for help again.

Q: *Will my therapist know if I don't do what they say I should?*

A: Therapists won't magically deduce that you haven't done your homework. Typically, they need to ask about it so that you can discuss it together. However, it tends to be clear to therapists when you have done your homework, since often that process will lead to other insights, thoughts, or observations.

Q: *How many sessions does it take to start feeling comfortable, really opening up, and sharing?*

A: That can depend. Part of it rests on how well you and your therapist "click" off the bat, which is where having a sense of shared identity (age, race, etc.) can be helpful, but not necessary. It also depends on how comfortable you feel in sharing about yourself generally. Another factor is the therapist's level of warmth. If you try sharing more than you typically might and the therapist's response helps put you at ease and makes you feel seen, then that is likely a good reinforcer for continuing to share.

Early indicators of whether this may be a setting where you could feel able to open up include a sense of feeling understood and respected, which can happen as early as in a phone consultation. Everyone experiences therapy differently, so it's important to observe when you start feeling safe and free to express yourself.

Q: *How do I know when therapy is working?*

A: While you want to give yourself and your therapist time to settle in and get to
know one another, it can be hard to know at what point you should start to see
results from your time together. Of course, if your goal was to change a behavior,
then an easy measure is whether you are able to do what you set out to do.
Otherwise, it can be helpful to reflect on your therapy goals and consider if the
things you were struggling with have more clarity or feel easier to engage with.
After you've been working for a little while, consider if there are any things that
have changed: how intense your feelings on something are, how you consider an
aspect of yourself, how you engage with others, how you respond to a situation.
These are signs that you have been integrating learnings from therapy into your
life. While things may not be quite where you want them to be, you are moving
in the right direction.

References

[1] Drisko, J. W. (2004). Common Factors in Psychotherapy Outcome: Meta-Analytic Findings and Their Implications for Practice and Research. Families in Society, 85(1), 81–90. ▸ https://doi.org/10.1606/1044-3894.239

[2] Norcross, JC, Wampold, BE. A new therapy for each patient: Evidence-based relationships and responsiveness. J. Clin. Psychol. 2018; 74: 1889– 1906.
▸ https://doi.org/10.1002/jclp.22678

[3] Stamoulos, C., Trepanier, L., Bourkas, S., Bradley, S., Stelmaszczyk, K., Schwartzman, D., & Drapeau, M. (2016). Psychologists' perceptions of the importance of common factors in psychotherapy for successful treatment outcomes. Journal of Psychotherapy Integration, 26(3), 300–317.
▸ https://doi.org/10.1037/a0040426

[4] Moors, F., & Zech, E. (2017). The Effects of Psychotherapist's and Clients' Interpersonal Behaviors during a First Simulated Session: A Lab Study Investigating Client Satisfaction. Frontiers in psychology, 8, 1868.
▸ https://doi.org/10.3389/fpsyg.2017.01868

[5] Ardito, R. B., & Rabellino, D. (2011). Therapeutic alliance and outcome of psychotherapy: historical excursus, measurements, and prospects for research. Frontiers in psychology, 2, 270. ▸ https://doi.org/10.3389/fpsyg.2011.00270

[6] Hatcher, R. L., & Barends, A. W. (2006). How a return to theory could help alliance research. Psychotherapy: Theory, Research, Practice, Training, 43(3), 292–299. ▸ https://doi.org/10.1037/0033-3204.43.3.292

[7] Eubanks, C. F., Muran, J. C., & Safran, J. D. (2019). Repairing alliance ruptures. In J. C. Norcross & M. J. Lambert (Eds.), Psychotherapy relationships that work: Evidence-based therapist contributions (pp. 549–579). Oxford University Press.
▸ https://doi.org/10.1093/med-psych/9780190843953.003.0016

[8] Krupnick, J. L., Sotsky, S. M., Elkin, I., Simmens, S., Moyer, J., Watkins, J., & Pilkonis, P. A. (2006). The Role of the Therapeutic Alliance in Psychotherapy and Pharmacotherapy Outcome: Findings in the National Institute of Mental Health Treatment of Depression Collaborative Research Program. FOCUS, 4(2), 269–277.
▸ https://doi.org/10.1176/foc.4.2.269

[9] Ardito, R. B., & Rabellino, D. (2011). Therapeutic alliance and outcome of psychotherapy: historical excursus, measurements, and prospects for research. Frontiers in psychology, 2, 270. ▸ https://doi.org/10.3389/fpsyg.2011.00270

[10] Dalle Grave R. (2020). Nutrition and Fitness: Mental Health. Nutrients, 12(6), 1804. ▸ https://doi.org/10.3390/nu12061804

[11] Ben Simon, E., Rossi, A., Harvey, A. G., & Walker, M. P. (2019). Overanxious and underslept. Nature Human Behaviour, 4(1), 100–110.
▸ https://doi.org/10.1038/s41562-019-0754-8

[12] Hölzel, B. K., Carmody, J., Vangel, M., Congleton, C., Yerramsetti, S. M., Gard, T., & Lazar, S. W. (2011). Mindfulness practice leads to increases in regional brain gray matter density. Psychiatry research, 191(1), 36–43.
▸ *https://doi.org/10.1016/j.pscychresns.2010.08.006*

[13] Holt-Lunstad, J., Smith, T. B., & Layton, J. B. (2010). Social relationships and mortality risk: a meta-analytic review. PLoS medicine, 7(7), e1000316.
▸ *https://doi.org/10.1371/journal.pmed.1000316*